Mediterranean Cortisol Reset for Women

A Stress-Lowering Diet to Balance Hormones, Burn Stubborn Belly Fat, Improve Sleep, and Restore Lasting Energy Naturally

Abigail Douglas

Contents

Preface

If you're holding this book, chances are you've tried to do everything "right."

You've eaten clean. You've cut calories. You've pushed through workouts. You've followed plans that promised to flatten your belly, boost your energy, and fix what felt off. And yet —despite your effort—you may still feel tired, wired at night, stuck with stubborn belly fat, battling cravings, or wondering why weight loss feels harder now than it used to.

This book begins with a different premise:

Your body is not broken. It's stressed.

For many women, especially in their 30s, 40s, 50s, and beyond, weight gain, poor sleep, low energy, and emotional eating are not signs of failure. They are signs of a stress response that has been running too long. Cortisol—the body's primary stress hormone—plays a central role in how we store fat, regulate appetite, manage blood sugar, and recover from daily life. When cortisol stays elevated, even the "healthiest" diet can stop working.

This is where the **Mediterranean Cortisol Reset for Women** comes in.

Unlike restrictive weight loss plans, extreme detoxes, or punishing routines, this approach is built around **stress-lowering nutrition, hormone balance, and metabolic safety**. It blends the science of cortisol regulation with the proven benefits of the Mediterranean diet—anti-inflammatory foods, balanced meals, healthy fats, and gentle rhythms that support long-term health.

Inside these pages, you'll learn why chronic stress quietly sabotages weight loss, sleep, and energy... why calorie restriction and over-exercising often make cortisol worse... and why women are especially sensitive to stress hormones during perimenopause, menopause, and high-demand seasons of life. More importantly, you'll learn what actually works.

This book offers a **practical 28-day cortisol reset plan** designed to stabilize blood sugar, calm the nervous system, support adrenal health, reduce cravings naturally, and help release stubborn belly fat without triggering stress spikes. You won't be asked to count calories, track macros, or eliminate entire food groups. Instead, you'll be guided toward Mediterranean meals that nourish rather than punish—meals that help you feel full, steady, and satisfied.

You'll also find strategies for real life: how to eat for calm energy instead of willpower, how to reduce emotional eating, how to improve sleep naturally, how to handle plateaus, and how to recover quickly when stress returns. The goal isn't perfection. It's **sustainable weight loss, steady energy, and a calm relationship with food**.

If you've been searching for a way to lose weight without constant hunger, stop cravings without restriction, improve sleep naturally, and feel normal around food again—this book was written for you. It's not another diet to follow temporarily. It's a framework you can return to whenever life gets loud.

This is an invitation to stop fighting your body and start supporting it.

Because when cortisol calms, everything else begins to work again.

Welcome to your reset—gentle, Mediterranean, and designed for women who are ready for relief, not rules.

Introduction

Your Body Is Not Broken—It's Stressed

If you've been eating "right," trying to move more, and still feel tired, puffy, restless at night, or stuck with stubborn belly fat, this book begins with a simple truth you may not have heard clearly before: **your body isn't failing you—it's protecting you**.

Stress hormones, especially cortisol, are designed to keep us alive. They sharpen focus, release fuel, and help us respond to danger. The problem isn't cortisol itself. The problem is **living in a world that never tells your body it's safe to turn cortisol off**. When stress becomes constant—deadlines, emotional load, poor sleep, undereating, overexercising—cortisol stops behaving like a helpful alarm and starts acting like a stuck switch. Weight loss slows. Sleep fractures. Energy drains. Cravings get louder. And the body, doing exactly what it's meant to do under threat, holds on.

Modern life quietly keeps cortisol "on" all the time. Screens before bed, caffeine replacing rest, rushed meals, skipped breakfasts, workouts that exhaust instead of restore—each one sends the same message to your nervous system: *stay alert*. For women, this message lands harder. Hormonal shifts across the menstrual cycle, perimenopause, and menopause make the stress response more sensitive. What once worked—cutting calories, pushing harder, ignoring hunger—often backfires now, amplifying the very symptoms you're trying to escape.

That's why extreme dieting feels so tempting and so punishing. It promises control, but it teaches your body scarcity. It asks for willpower when what your system is craving is stability. The result is a cycle of effort and exhaustion: short bursts of progress followed by stalls, rebounds, and self-blame. This book breaks that cycle by changing the question from *"How do I force my body to lose weight?"* to *"How do I help my body feel safe enough to let go?"*

The Mediterranean way offers a different answer—one rooted in calm, nourishment, and longevity. This isn't a list of forbidden foods or a rigid plan to follow perfectly. It's a pattern of eating and living that lowers inflammation, steadies blood sugar, supports gut health, and sends repeated signals of safety to the nervous system. Real food, eaten regularly. Healthy fats that satisfy. Carbohydrates without fear. Protein timed to support energy, not punish hunger. Over time, these choices quiet cortisol's constant hum and allow the body to return to balance.

Over the next 28 days, you'll gently reset the systems stress disrupts most: blood sugar, sleep rhythms, appetite cues, energy flow, and fat storage patterns. Not through punishment, restriction, or obsession—but through consistency, nourishment, and trust. You won't be asked to track every bite, push through exhaustion, or ignore your body's signals. Instead, you'll learn how to work with them. As cortisol settles, many women notice better sleep, calmer cravings, steadier energy, and a body that finally feels willing to respond.

This is not about fixing yourself. It's about creating the conditions your body has been asking for all along.

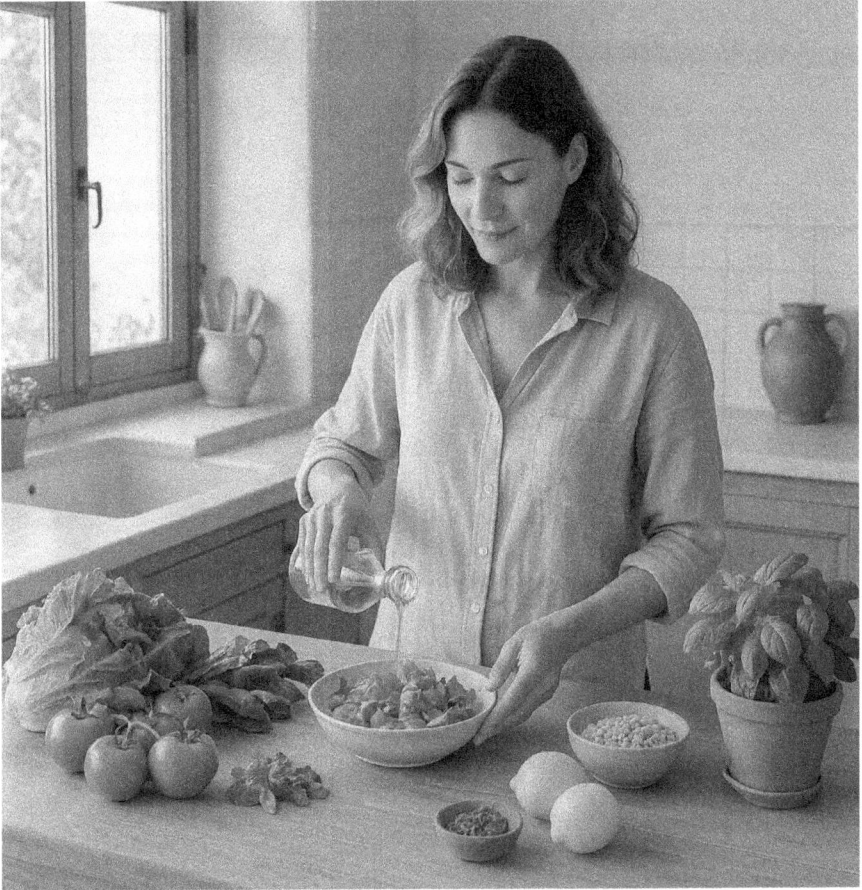

PART I — UNDERSTANDING CORTISOL & THE FEMALE BODY

Chapter 1

Cortisol Explained in Human Language

Cortisol has earned a bad reputation. In wellness headlines and social media clips, it's often painted as the villain behind stubborn belly fat, sleepless nights, and relentless cravings. But cortisol is not your enemy. In fact, without it, you wouldn't get out of bed, think clearly, or respond to danger. The problem isn't cortisol itself—it's **how often your body is being asked to produce it, and whether it ever gets the message that it's safe to stand down**.

This chapter strips cortisol of its mystery and fear. No medical jargon. No blame. Just a clear understanding of what cortisol does, why women are especially sensitive to it, and how a constantly "on" stress response quietly reshapes the body over time.

What Cortisol Really Does (and Why You Need It)

Cortisol is your body's primary **stress-response hormone**. It's produced by the adrenal glands and released when your brain senses a need for alertness or action. Think of cortisol as an internal manager. When it rises at the right time and in the right amount, it helps you:

- Wake up in the morning

- Mobilize energy so you can think and move

- Regulate blood sugar between meals

- Reduce inflammation after injury

- Handle short-term challenges

In a healthy rhythm, cortisol follows a daily pattern. It rises in the early morning to help you feel alert, gradually declines throughout the day, and reaches its lowest point at night so your body can rest, repair, and sleep deeply.

This rhythm is essential. Cortisol isn't meant to be eliminated—it's meant to be **balanced**.

Problems begin when cortisol stops following this natural rise-and-fall pattern and instead stays elevated, erratic, or suppressed at the wrong times. That's when its helpful functions turn disruptive.

Acute Stress vs. Chronic Stress: The Difference That Matters

Your body was designed to handle **acute stress**. A near accident, a sudden loud noise, an urgent deadline—these moments trigger a temporary cortisol spike. Once the situation passes, cortisol drops, and the body returns to baseline. This is healthy. It's protective.

Chronic stress, however, is different. It's not one dramatic moment—it's a steady stream of pressures that never fully resolve. Think:

- Skipping meals or eating on the run

- Sleeping poorly night after night

- Overexercising while undereating

- Emotional strain, caregiving, financial worry

- Constant notifications, noise, and stimulation

- Dieting that keeps the body in perceived scarcity

Under chronic stress, cortisol doesn't get the "all clear" signal. The body remains in a low-grade state of alert. Over time, this changes how your metabolism works, how fat is stored, how hunger signals behave, and how well you sleep.

Your body isn't overreacting—it's **adapting**.

Why Women Are More Cortisol-Sensitive

Women's bodies are exquisitely responsive systems. Estrogen, progesterone, insulin, thyroid hormones, and cortisol all communicate with one another. When one becomes dysregulated, the effects ripple outward.

Several factors make women more sensitive to cortisol disruption:

- **Hormonal fluctuations** across the menstrual cycle

- **Perimenopause and menopause**, when estrogen declines and stress tolerance narrows

- **Lower muscle mass**, which affects glucose storage and stress recovery

- **Cultural pressure** to diet, restrict, and push through fatigue

- **Emotional labor**, which the nervous system registers as real stress

As estrogen changes, cortisol's impact intensifies. What once felt manageable may suddenly feel overwhelming. Sleep becomes lighter. Recovery takes longer. Weight loss strategies that worked in the past stop working—or make things worse.

This isn't weakness. It's biology.

When cortisol remains elevated, women's bodies often choose **protection over progress**. Fat loss slows. Appetite cues become confusing. Energy dips. The body prioritizes survival, not aesthetics.

Cortisol's Link to Belly Fat, Cravings, and Inflammation

Cortisol has a special relationship with abdominal fat. Fat cells in the belly area contain more cortisol receptors than fat cells elsewhere. When cortisol stays high, the body preferentially stores energy in this region because it's close to vital organs and easily accessible in an emergency.

This is why belly fat can feel so stubborn—even when you're eating well and exercising.

Cortisol also affects **blood sugar regulation**. When it rises, it signals the liver to release glucose into the bloodstream. If this happens too often, blood sugar becomes unstable, leading to:

- Energy crashes

- Intense cravings, especially for sugar and refined carbs

- Irritability and anxiety when meals are delayed

- Late-night hunger

Over time, chronic cortisol elevation promotes **low-grade inflammation**. This inflammation isn't always painful or obvious, but it interferes with insulin sensitivity, digestion, joint comfort, and immune resilience. The body feels "puffy," reactive, and slow to recover.

Again, these are not signs of failure. They are signs of a body under prolonged pressure.

Signs Your Cortisol Rhythm Is Disrupted

Cortisol imbalance doesn't look the same for everyone. Some women have cortisol that's consistently high; others have cortisol that's low when it should be high (like in the morning) and elevated at night. Both patterns are disruptive.

Common signs include:

- Feeling tired but wired

- Difficulty falling or staying asleep

- Waking up exhausted despite adequate sleep time

- Cravings that feel urgent rather than optional

- Weight gain concentrated around the midsection

- Anxiety or restlessness without a clear cause

- Needing caffeine to function

- Feeling worse when you diet harder or exercise more

If you recognize yourself in this list, the answer isn't more discipline. It's **more safety**—physiological, emotional, and nutritional.

That's where the Mediterranean cortisol reset begins. By stabilizing blood sugar, providing consistent nourishment, lowering inflammation, and restoring daily rhythm, the body receives a new message: *you are not under threat*. When that message is repeated often enough, cortisol settles, and the body becomes willing to change again.

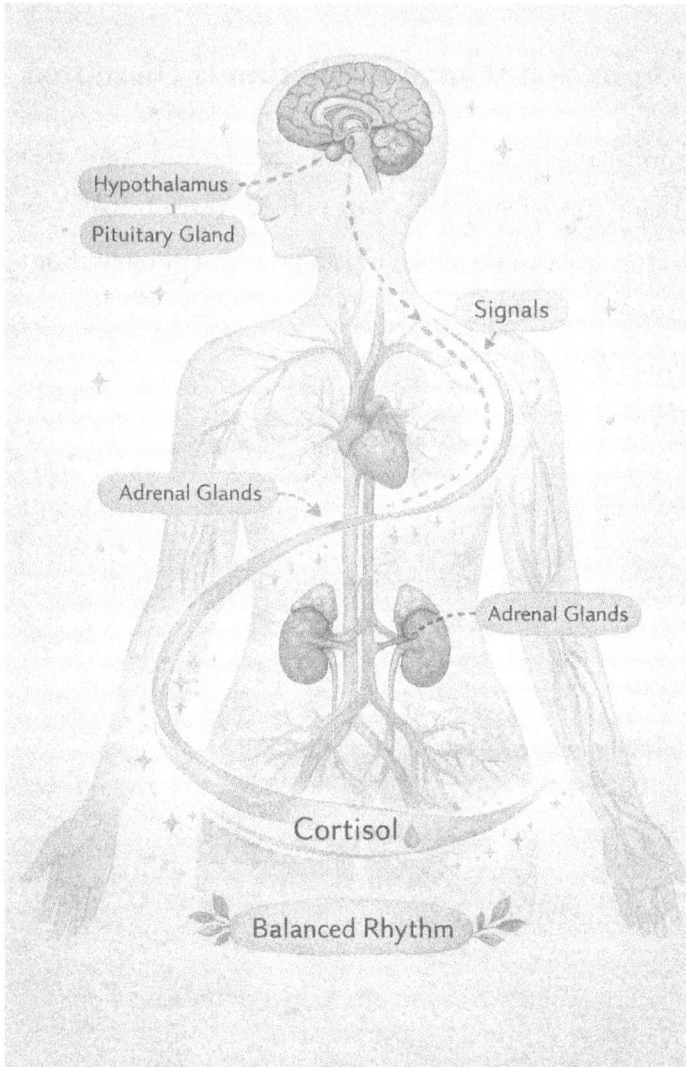

Chapter 2

Why Dieting Makes Stress Worse for Women

When it comes to stress, dieting can often make things worse. While the intention behind most diet plans is to promote health and fat loss, they inadvertently trigger a physiological response that raises cortisol, the body's primary stress hormone. If you've ever felt more anxious, drained, or irritable while trying to lose weight, you're not alone. It's not just about willpower—it's about biology.

Calorie Restriction and Cortisol Spikes

In simple terms, when your body feels like it's not getting enough energy (calories), it responds by producing more cortisol. Cortisol's primary job is to keep you alive under stress, and one of its roles is to release stored energy (in the form of glucose) to keep you going. However, when calories are restricted for too long, cortisol stays high, which can lead to several issues:

- **Fat storage**: While cortisol mobilizes energy, it also signals the body to store fat, especially around the belly. This is a survival mechanism, as the body perceives scarcity and holds onto resources.

- **Increased cravings**: High cortisol leads to cravings, particularly for sugary, high-carb foods that provide quick energy.

- **Fatigue and burnout**: The body is in a constant state of alert, which leads to exhaustion over time. Your body's stress response works overtime, and you feel the effects in both your mental and physical energy levels.

When calorie restriction is too severe or prolonged, cortisol doesn't get a break. Instead of weight loss, you're left with increased stress, weight plateaus, and frustrated attempts at control.

Over-Exercising and Under-Eating

Much like extreme calorie restriction, over-exercising while under-eating compounds the effects of high cortisol. Women, especially, have a unique hormonal profile that makes them more sensitive to the stresses of high-intensity exercise, especially when combined with insufficient nutrition.

This scenario is all too common for women who are trying to burn fat through excessive workouts without properly fueling their bodies. While exercise is healthy, pushing the body too hard without enough nutrients or rest leads to:

- **Chronic cortisol elevation**: More physical stress from over-exercising means more cortisol, which, in turn, makes fat loss harder and fatigue more pronounced.

- **Impaired recovery**: Without proper rest and nutrition, the body can't effectively recover from the physical stress of intense workouts. This results in muscle depletion rather than fat loss, further slowing your metabolism.

- **Increased cravings**: Over-exercising increases hunger, but the body will crave quick sources of fuel (sugar, refined carbs), which further heightens cortisol levels.

When the body is in a constant state of stress due to over-exercising and under-eating, it enters a fight-or-flight mode, rather than a fat-burning or recovery mode. This makes fat loss not only harder but potentially impossible.

Blood Sugar Crashes and Anxiety

One of cortisol's primary functions is to regulate blood sugar levels, but when your body is chronically stressed, it begins to overproduce glucose to provide energy in times of perceived danger. When blood sugar is unstable, it can lead to sharp fluctuations that cause:

- **Blood sugar crashes**: After a spike in blood sugar, your body releases insulin to lower it, which can then cause a sudden dip, leaving you feeling irritable, anxious, and fatigued.

- **Anxiety**: Low blood sugar levels activate the fight-or-flight response, raising cortisol and causing feelings of stress and anxiety. When blood sugar dips too low, it fuels the cycle of stress and anxiety, leading to more cravings for sugary foods to bring levels back up.

A constant cycle of blood sugar spikes and crashes, paired with the stress hormone cortisol, creates a feeling of nervous energy and emotional turbulence. This cycle makes it harder for the body to properly metabolize fat and restore hormonal balance.

Why "Discipline" Isn't the Solution

One of the biggest myths in the dieting world is the idea that **discipline** is the solution to weight loss. We've been taught that the harder you push yourself, the more successful you'll be. But for women, particularly those dealing with stress, this mindset is counterproductive.

The issue with the "discipline" approach is that it often leads to **restrictive eating**, **extreme workouts**, and **emotional burnout**. Instead of seeing discipline as a way to control the body, it's better to see it as a way to nourish it—**through steady, consistent habits** that focus on long-term wellness rather than short-term willpower.

Pushing through fatigue, skipping meals, or continuing to exercise through exhaustion may seem like an act of discipline, but it's actually stressing your body out more and keeping cortisol levels elevated. This only leads to weight stalls, emotional exhaustion, and heightened stress responses.

The Safety-First Approach to Fat Loss

The key to sustainable, healthy fat loss is adopting a **safety-first approach**. Instead of pushing the body beyond its limits, a safer approach nourishes the body, stabilizes blood sugar, and calms the stress response. Here's how to do it:

- **Eat consistently**: Rather than restricting food, focus on consistent meals and snacks that stabilize blood sugar and provide steady energy throughout the day.

- **Prioritize recovery**: Rest is just as important as exercise. Focus on sleep, gentle movement, and stress reduction to help your body recover.

- **Listen to your body**: Trust your body's hunger and fullness cues. Let your body guide you rather than forcing it to comply with an external "diet."

- **Include cortisol-calming foods**: Foods rich in healthy fats (like olive oil, avocado, nuts), lean proteins, and fiber (like vegetables and whole grains) help stabilize blood sugar and support hormonal balance.

By focusing on nourishment, rest, and balanced exercise, your body can return to a state of **safety**—and when the body feels safe, it's finally willing to release stored fat.

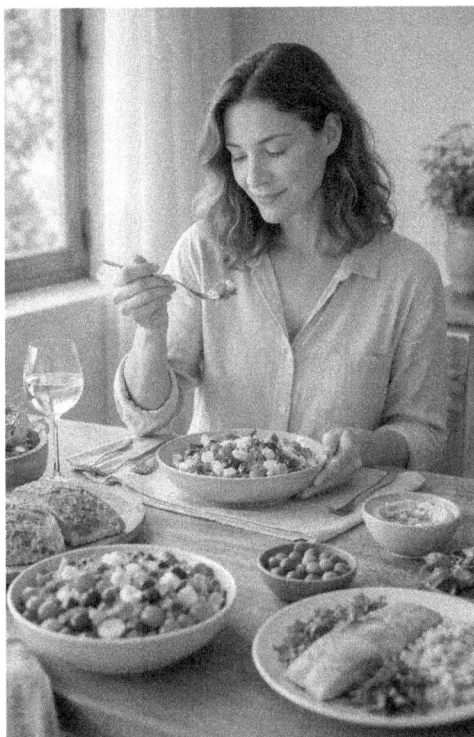

Chapter 3

The Mediterranean Advantage for Hormone Balance

B y now, you understand that cortisol doesn't misbehave on its own—it responds to signals. Food is one of the strongest signals your body receives every single day. Not just *what* you eat, but *how often*, *how consistently*, and *in what context*. This is where the Mediterranean way quietly outperforms almost every modern diet, especially for women under stress.

The Mediterranean pattern wasn't designed for weight loss trends or metabolic hacks. It evolved over generations to support **resilience, recovery, and longevity**. And those are precisely the conditions cortisol needs to settle.

Why This Eating Pattern Lowers Inflammation

Chronic inflammation and chronic stress are deeply intertwined. When inflammation rises, cortisol often follows—attempting to manage damage and restore balance. The Mediterranean way naturally lowers this inflammatory burden without aggressive rules or restriction.

This happens because the diet emphasizes foods that *calm* the immune system rather than provoke it. Vegetables, fruits, legumes, herbs, olive oil, fish, and whole grains provide a steady supply of anti-inflammatory compounds that reduce oxidative stress in the body. At the same time, highly processed foods—those most likely to trigger inflammation and blood sugar chaos—are naturally minimized, not forbidden.

What matters most is consistency. Inflammation doesn't drop because of one "perfect" meal. It eases when the body repeatedly receives the message that nourishment is reliable and gentle. Over time, this reduces the need for cortisol to stay elevated as a protective response.

Fiber, Fats, and Antioxidants—Explained Simply

You don't need to memorize nutrients to benefit from them. The Mediterranean advantage comes down to three core elements working together.

Fiber acts like a stabilizer. It slows digestion, steadies blood sugar, feeds beneficial gut bacteria, and reduces the sharp glucose swings that trigger cortisol release. When meals are fiber-rich, the body doesn't feel rushed or threatened—it feels supported.

Healthy fats, especially from olive oil, nuts, seeds, and fish, signal safety. Fat slows the absorption of carbohydrates, improves satiety, and supports hormone production. For women, dietary fat is not optional—it's foundational. Adequate fat intake helps regulate appetite hormones and reduces the stress response associated with under-eating.

Antioxidants—found in colorful plants, herbs, spices, and extra-virgin olive oil—quiet cellular stress. They help neutralize the internal "noise" created by pollution, poor sleep, emotional strain, and inflammation. When oxidative stress drops, cortisol no longer needs to act as a constant firefighter.

Together, these elements create meals that feel grounding instead of stimulating, satisfying instead of activating.

How Mediterranean Eating Supports Adrenal Recovery

Your adrenal glands don't burn out overnight. They become strained when they're repeatedly asked to respond to emergencies that never end. Mediterranean-style eating helps reverse this strain by restoring rhythm.

Regular meals prevent blood sugar emergencies. Adequate protein supports tissue repair. Healthy fats provide long-lasting energy. Micronutrients from whole foods replenish what stress depletes—magnesium, potassium, B vitamins, and antioxidants that support adrenal signaling.

Just as important, Mediterranean eating removes the *pressure* of perfection. There's no countdown clock between meals. No fear of combining foods incorrectly. No demand to push through hunger. That psychological safety matters. When food stops feeling like a threat or a test, cortisol has one less reason to stay elevated.

Recovery doesn't happen because the adrenals are "stimulated." It happens because they're finally allowed to rest.

The Role of Gut Health in Cortisol Regulation

Your gut and your stress hormones are in constant conversation. The gut communicates with the brain through nerves, immune signals, and chemical messengers. When gut health is compromised, the brain often interprets it as danger—and cortisol rises accordingly.

The Mediterranean pattern supports gut health naturally. Fiber feeds beneficial bacteria. Fermented foods encourage microbial diversity. Polyphenols from olive oil, vegetables, and herbs help maintain the gut lining. Together, these reduce intestinal irritation and inflammation.

A healthier gut sends calmer signals to the brain. That means fewer false alarms, less background anxiety, and a more stable cortisol rhythm. Over time, digestion improves, bloating decreases, and food becomes easier to tolerate—another sign that the body is shifting out of survival mode.

Longevity Data Women Can Trust

The Mediterranean lifestyle is one of the most studied eating patterns in the world—not for short-term weight loss, but for **long-term health**. Populations that follow it consistently show lower rates of heart disease, metabolic disorders, cognitive decline, and chronic inflammation.

For women, this matters deeply. Longevity isn't just about living longer—it's about maintaining energy, mobility, clarity, and independence as hormones change. Diets that rely on restriction often worsen stress over time. The Mediterranean approach does the opposite: it becomes more supportive as the body ages.

What the data consistently shows is this: eating in a way that lowers inflammation, stabilizes blood sugar, and supports social connection leads to better outcomes—not just physically, but emotionally and hormonally. That's why this approach doesn't fight cortisol. It **outgrows the need for it to stay elevated**.

The Mediterranean advantage isn't willpower. It's wisdom—applied gently, repeatedly, and with trust in the body's capacity to heal when the environment supports it.

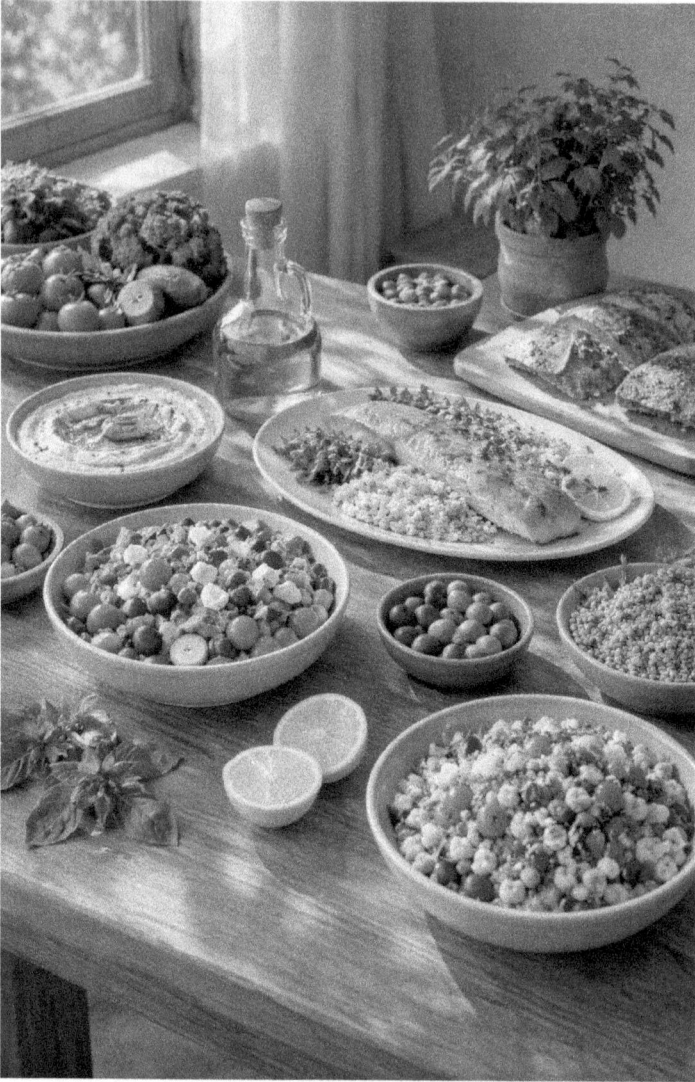

PART II — THE CORTISOL RESET PRINCIPLES

Chapter 4

The Non-Negotiables of a Cortisol-Calming Diet

W hen cortisol is stuck on high alert, the body becomes less responsive to effort and more protective of its resources. That's why random "healthy choices" don't always translate into better results. A cortisol-calming diet isn't about eating perfectly—it's about meeting a few **non-negotiable needs** that tell your nervous system it's safe to stand down.

These principles are simple, but they're powerful. When practiced consistently, they create the internal conditions that allow hormones to rebalance, energy to return, and fat loss to feel possible again.

Stable Blood Sugar Basics

Blood sugar stability is the foundation of cortisol balance. Every sharp rise or crash in blood sugar is interpreted by the body as a stress event. When that happens, cortisol steps in to manage the crisis by releasing stored glucose. If these swings happen repeatedly throughout the day, cortisol never gets a break.

A cortisol-calming diet focuses on **steady fuel**, not peaks and valleys. That means:

- Eating regular meals instead of skipping and "catching up later"

- Pairing carbohydrates with protein, fat, or fiber

- Avoiding long stretches of hunger that trigger adrenaline and cortisol

Stable blood sugar creates predictable energy. Predictability is calming to the nervous system. Over time, this steadiness reduces cravings, improves mood, and lowers the background stress load the body carries all day.

Protein Timing for Women

Protein matters—but timing matters just as much, especially for women.

Many women under-eat protein earlier in the day and then try to compensate at dinner. From a cortisol perspective, this pattern is stressful. Morning and midday are when cortisol is naturally higher. Without enough protein at these times, blood sugar drops faster, and cortisol rises further to compensate.

A cortisol-calming approach prioritizes **earlier protein intake**:

- Protein at breakfast helps blunt the morning cortisol spike

- Protein at lunch supports sustained energy and focus

- Adequate protein throughout the day reduces late-day cravings

This isn't about eating large portions. It's about giving your body the amino acids it needs when it needs them, so cortisol doesn't have to keep stepping in as a backup system.

Healthy Fats That Signal Safety to the Body

Dietary fat has been misunderstood for decades, but from a hormonal perspective, it's one of the most calming nutrients you can eat.

Healthy fats slow digestion, support satiety, and stabilize blood sugar. More importantly, they send a powerful signal of **abundance**, not scarcity. When the body senses adequate fat intake, it relaxes its grip on stored energy.

Mediterranean fats—olive oil, nuts, seeds, fatty fish, olives, and avocado—are especially supportive because they:

- Reduce inflammation

- Improve insulin sensitivity

- Support hormone production

- Help meals feel satisfying instead of rushed

When fat is consistently included, cortisol doesn't need to stay elevated to "protect" energy reserves.

Carbs Without Fear (and Without Spikes)

Carbohydrates are not the enemy of cortisol balance. In fact, overly restricting carbs can raise cortisol, disrupt sleep, and intensify cravings—especially in women.

The key is **carb quality and context**.

Whole, fiber-rich carbohydrates—vegetables, legumes, fruits, and whole grains—digest more slowly and feed the gut microbiome. When eaten with protein and fat, they provide steady glucose instead of sharp spikes.

A cortisol-calming diet allows carbs without guilt, because:

- Carbs help lower cortisol after stress

- Adequate carbs support serotonin and sleep

- Fear around food is itself a stress signal

When carbs are eaten calmly, consistently, and without restriction, the body stops reacting defensively to them.

Foods That Quietly Raise Cortisol

Not all cortisol triggers feel dramatic. Some foods raise cortisol subtly, over time, by stressing blood sugar, digestion, or the nervous system.

Common examples include:

- Highly refined sugars eaten alone

- Ultra-processed foods with little fiber or protein

- Excess caffeine, especially on an empty stomach

- Alcohol used frequently to "relax"

- Long periods of under-eating followed by overeating

These foods aren't moral failures. They simply add to the body's stress load when consumed frequently or without balance. The goal isn't elimination—it's awareness and context.

When nourishing foods become the default, these cortisol-raising foods naturally lose their grip.

The Bigger Picture

A cortisol-calming diet isn't rigid. It doesn't demand perfection. Its power lies in **reliability**.

When meals are regular, balanced, and satisfying, the body learns that energy is available and danger has passed. Cortisol lowers not because you force it to—but because it's no longer needed.

That's when the body begins to cooperate again.

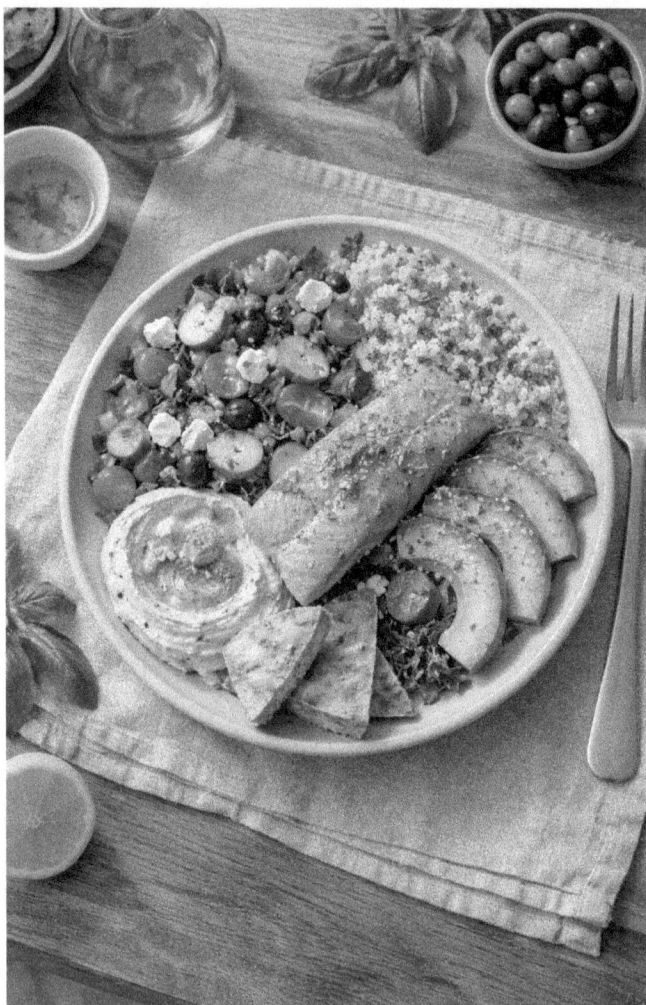

Chapter 5

Eating for Calm Energy, Not Willpower

For many women, eating has become an act of management—controlling portions, fighting cravings, overriding hunger, negotiating guilt. All of that effort requires willpower, and willpower is expensive. It draws on the same stress systems that cortisol already keeps busy. When food choices rely on constant self-control, the body stays tense, alert, and guarded.

Calm energy comes from a different place. It comes from learning how to eat in a way that *reduces* internal noise instead of adding to it—so the body doesn't need discipline to cooperate.

Hunger vs. Stress Cravings

True hunger is physical. It builds gradually. It's often felt in the stomach, the body, the energy level. Stress cravings, on the other hand, are urgent and specific. They arrive suddenly. They demand quick relief—usually sugar, salt, or something crunchy.

Cortisol plays a central role here. When stress is high or blood sugar drops, cortisol signals the brain to seek fast fuel. That signal can feel indistinguishable from hunger, especially if you've been dieting, skipping meals, or running on caffeine.

Learning the difference isn't about resisting cravings. It's about *preventing* them by meeting your body's needs earlier:

- Regular meals reduce cortisol-driven urgency

- Balanced plates stabilize blood sugar

- Adequate carbohydrates reduce the "emergency" signal

When the body trusts that nourishment is coming, cravings soften. They stop shouting because they no longer need to.

The Psychology of "Enough"

Diet culture teaches us to stop eating based on rules—calories, portions, points. A cortisol-calming approach teaches you to stop eating based on **sufficiency**.

"Enough" isn't a number. It's a sensation. It's the moment when hunger fades, breathing slows, and the body settles. For many women, this signal has been drowned out by years of restriction and urgency.

Psychologically, the body needs permission to believe food will be available again. When meals are consistent and satisfying, the nervous system relaxes. Eating becomes less frantic. Stopping feels natural instead of forced.

Enough is not deprivation. It's completion.

Portion Awareness Without Tracking

Tracking portions can be helpful short-term, but long-term reliance on measuring keeps the brain in evaluation mode. Evaluation is stressful. It keeps cortisol engaged.

Portion awareness without tracking is about *visual balance* and *internal feedback*:

- A source of protein at each meal

- Generous vegetables or fiber-rich plants

- Healthy fats for satisfaction

- Carbohydrates included intentionally, not avoided

When meals are built this way, the body self-regulates more easily. You don't need to calculate when your plate already communicates balance.

This approach removes pressure. And pressure is one of the fastest ways to keep cortisol elevated.

Gentle Satiety Cues Women Can Trust

Satiety doesn't arrive as a hard stop. It's subtle, especially in women whose stress response has been active for years. Learning to notice it requires slowing down—not dramatically, just enough to check in.

Common satiety cues include:

- Food starts tasting less intense

- Breathing deepens

- Shoulders relax

- The urge to keep eating fades

- A sense of comfort replaces urgency

These cues are easiest to notice when meals aren't rushed and hunger isn't extreme. That's why regular eating matters. When you arrive at meals overly hungry, cortisol is already elevated, and satiety signals get delayed.

Trust builds when you respond to these cues consistently. Over time, the body learns you're listening—and it responds with steadier appetite regulation.

How to Stop Eating Without Guilt

Guilt keeps cortisol high. It frames eating as a moral act instead of a biological one. When guilt enters the picture, even a nourishing meal becomes stressful.

Stopping without guilt begins with understanding this: **eating enough is not overeating**. It's information. It tells the body it can relax.

If you stop eating because you feel satisfied—not because you've hit a limit—you've completed the meal. No apology required. No compensation later. No mental tally.

When guilt is removed, cortisol lowers. When cortisol lowers, appetite regulation improves. And when appetite regulation improves, willpower becomes unnecessary.

The Shift That Changes Everything

Eating for calm energy is not about eating less. It's about eating in a way that *costs less stress*. When meals provide stability, reassurance, and satisfaction, the body stops bracing itself.

And when the body stops bracing, energy returns—not as a spike, but as a steady, livable flow.

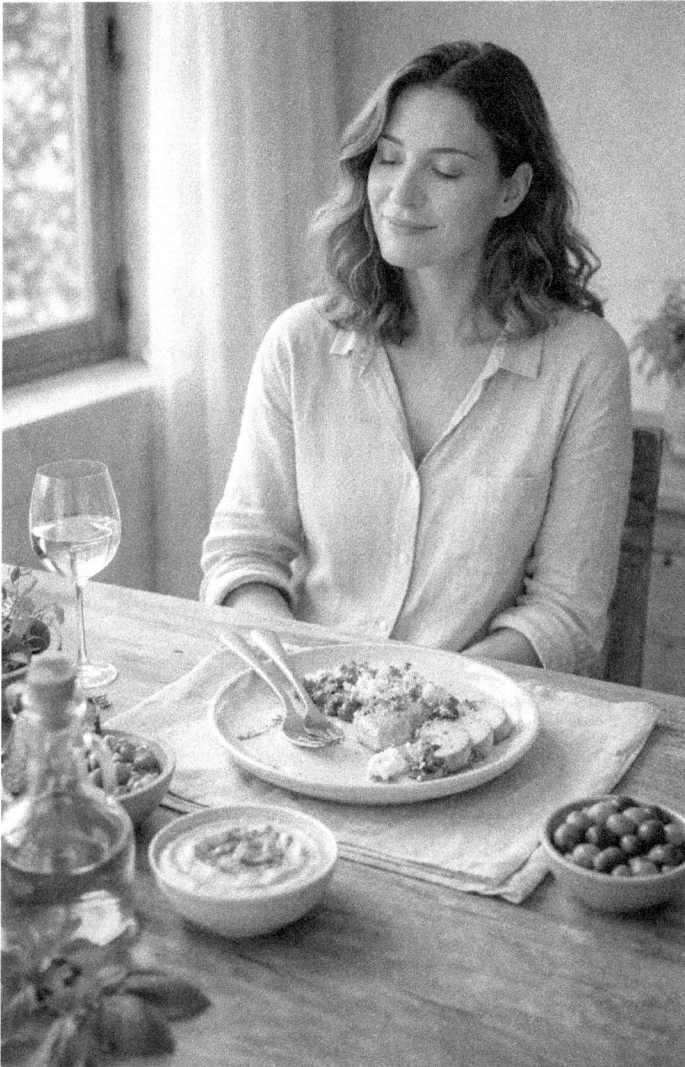

Chapter 6

Lifestyle Habits That Make the Diet Work

F ood sets the foundation, but lifestyle determines whether that foundation holds. You can eat beautifully and still feel wired, tired, or stuck if your daily rhythms continue to signal urgency to your nervous system. Cortisol responds not just to what's on your plate, but to **how you wake, move, rest, stimulate, and emotionally carry your days**.

This chapter brings the diet to life. These habits don't require perfection or major upheaval. They work because they're small, repeatable, and biologically meaningful—quiet signals that tell your body it's safe to shift out of survival mode.

Sleep Timing and Cortisol Rhythm

Cortisol and sleep are inseparable partners. In a healthy rhythm, cortisol peaks in the early morning to help you wake and declines throughout the day, reaching its lowest point at night so sleep can deepen and repair can occur.

When sleep is delayed, fragmented, or inconsistent, this rhythm breaks down. Cortisol may stay elevated late into the evening, making it hard to fall asleep. Or it may drop too low in the morning, leaving you groggy and dependent on caffeine.

What matters most isn't perfect sleep—it's **predictable sleep timing**. Going to bed and waking up around the same time each day trains your nervous system to expect rest. Even modest consistency helps cortisol re-learn its natural curve.

Simple adjustments that support this rhythm:

- A gentle wind-down routine that signals the day is ending

- Dimming lights in the evening

- Avoiding stimulating tasks late at night

- Letting sleep be restorative, not something to "optimize"

Sleep doesn't need to be forced. It needs to be invited.

Morning Light Exposure

One of the most powerful cortisol regulators costs nothing: **natural morning light**.

When light enters your eyes early in the day, it sends a signal to the brain that it's time to set the day's hormonal rhythm. Cortisol rises appropriately, melatonin lowers, and your internal clock aligns with the environment.

This doesn't require sunbathing or long walks. A few minutes near a window, stepping outside briefly, or opening curtains soon after waking is enough to anchor your circadian rhythm.

Consistent morning light:

- Improves daytime energy

- Supports nighttime sleep

- Reduces late-night cortisol spikes

- Helps regulate appetite timing

It's a gentle reset, repeated daily.

Caffeine and Cortisol: What to Adjust

Caffeine isn't inherently harmful—but timing and context matter, especially when cortisol is already strained.

Caffeine stimulates cortisol release. When consumed first thing in the morning, especially on an empty stomach, it can exaggerate the natural cortisol peak and contribute to anxiety, jitters, or mid-morning crashes.

A cortisol-calming approach doesn't demand elimination. It invites **strategic use**:

- Eat before or with caffeine when possible

- Delay caffeine slightly after waking

- Notice how much supports energy versus overstimulation

- Consider reducing caffeine during high-stress periods

The goal isn't deprivation. It's cooperation. When caffeine works *with* your rhythm instead of against it, energy becomes steadier and calmer.

Gentle Movement vs. Intense Workouts

Movement is essential—but not all movement communicates safety.

High-intensity exercise, especially when paired with under-eating or poor sleep, can act as another stressor. Cortisol rises to meet the demand, recovery slows, and fat loss may stall despite effort.

Gentle, rhythmic movement sends a different message. Walking, stretching, mobility work, light strength training, and restorative practices support circulation and insulin sensitivity without triggering a stress response.

This doesn't mean intense workouts are forbidden. It means they should be:

- Appropriately fueled

- Balanced with recovery

- Matched to your current stress capacity

The body responds best when movement energizes rather than depletes. Progress happens when cortisol isn't constantly called in to manage exhaustion.

Emotional Stress and Food Choices

Emotional stress is real stress. The nervous system doesn't distinguish between an emotional burden and a physical threat. When emotional load increases, cortisol rises—and food choices shift accordingly.

Under stress, the brain seeks quick comfort and fast energy. This isn't a failure of discipline. It's a biological response to perceived threat.

What helps isn't restriction—it's **compassion and structure**:

- Regular meals reduce emotional eating urgency

- Balanced nutrition lowers reactivity

- Gentle routines create emotional containment

- Self-judgment raises cortisol; self-trust lowers it

Food becomes calmer when life feels more supported. And life feels more supported when small rituals—meals, movement, rest—are predictable and kind.

Bringing It All Together

These habits don't work because they're impressive. They work because they're **reassuring**.

Each one repeats the same message: you are safe, you are nourished, you are allowed to rest.

When that message is heard often enough, cortisol no longer needs to stay on guard. The diet begins to work not through effort, but through alignment.

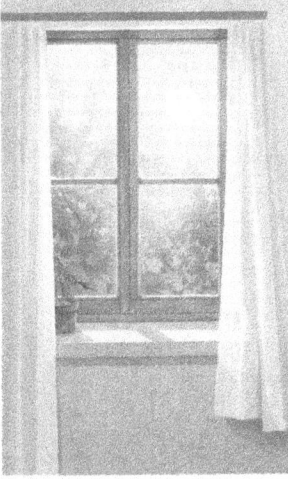
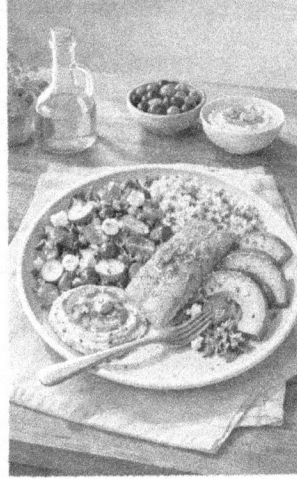
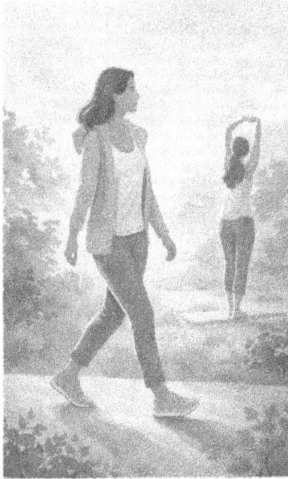
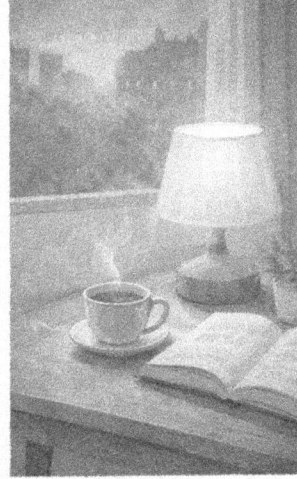

PART III — THE 28-DAY MEDITERRANEAN CORTISOL RESET

Chapter 7

How to Use the 28-Day Reset

T his reset is not a test of discipline. It's not a challenge to "be good," eat perfectly, or push through discomfort. It's a **physiological re-calibration**—a structured period of nourishment and rhythm designed to help your nervous system stand down and your hormones begin to cooperate again.

How you approach these 28 days matters as much as what you eat. This chapter shows you exactly what to expect, what to avoid, and how to adapt the reset to your real life without undoing its benefits.

What Changes to Expect Week by Week

Cortisol doesn't reset overnight. It responds to **repeated signals of safety**, and those signals accumulate gradually.

Week 1: Stabilization

This week is about calming blood sugar and reducing internal urgency. You may notice:

- Hunger becoming more predictable

- Fewer extreme cravings

- Mild fatigue as your body shifts out of constant alert

- Improved digestion or reduced bloating

Emotionally, this week can feel grounding—or surprisingly emotional. That's normal. As cortisol lowers, awareness increases.

Week 2: Calming the Stress Response

Sleep often begins to improve here. Energy becomes steadier rather than spiky. Cravings lose intensity. You may feel calmer during the day and less wired at night.

This is when many women realize how much background stress they were carrying.

Week 3: Gentle Release

This is where stubborn belly fat may start to respond—not because you're trying harder, but because the body feels safer letting go. Appetite cues feel clearer. You may notice changes in how clothes fit or how your body feels after meals.

The scale may fluctuate. That's normal. Focus on signals, not numbers.

Week 4: Restoration and Momentum

Energy feels more reliable. Food decisions feel less charged. You're no longer "managing" yourself around meals—you're responding. This week is about confidence and sustainability, not pushing for dramatic change.

How Hunger, Energy, and Sleep May Shift

Hunger often becomes **more honest** during this reset. At first, you may feel hungrier than expected—this is your body testing whether nourishment is reliable. Responding consistently helps cortisol settle.

Energy shifts from sharp bursts to a steadier flow. Instead of needing caffeine to function, you may notice fewer crashes and more mental clarity.

Sleep may improve gradually. Falling asleep can become easier before staying asleep does. That's still progress. Cortisol rhythms repair in layers. All of these shifts are signs of recalibration, not failure.

What *Not* to Do During the Reset

This reset works best when it's **protected from extremes**. Avoid:

- Skipping meals to "speed things up"

- Adding intense workouts without adequate fuel

- Cutting carbs out of fear

- Tracking calories obsessively

- Comparing your progress to anyone else's

These behaviors send mixed signals to your nervous system. Consistency—not intensity—is what lowers cortisol.

How to Personalize Without Sabotaging Results

Personalization is encouraged. Chaos is not.

You can adapt the reset by:

- Swapping proteins or vegetables you prefer

- Adjusting meal timing to fit your schedule

- Eating more if hunger persists

- Choosing gentler movement when stressed

What matters is keeping the **core signals intact**: regular meals, balanced plates, adequate rest, and emotional neutrality around food.

Personalization works when it's rooted in listening, not control.

Safety Notes for Women Over 40

As estrogen declines, stress tolerance narrows. That means your body may respond more strongly—both positively and negatively—to changes.

Important reminders:

- Eat enough, especially protein and carbohydrates

- Prioritize sleep over aggressive exercise

- Expect slower but more sustainable fat loss

- Listen for fatigue rather than pushing through it

If you have medical conditions, are on medication, or have a history of disordered eating, this reset should be approached gently and with professional guidance if needed.

The goal is support, not strain.

The Right Mindset for These 28 Days

Think of this reset as **practice**, not performance. You're teaching your body a new rhythm—one where nourishment is steady, stress is reduced, and cortisol no longer needs to stay on guard.

When that rhythm becomes familiar, change happens naturally.

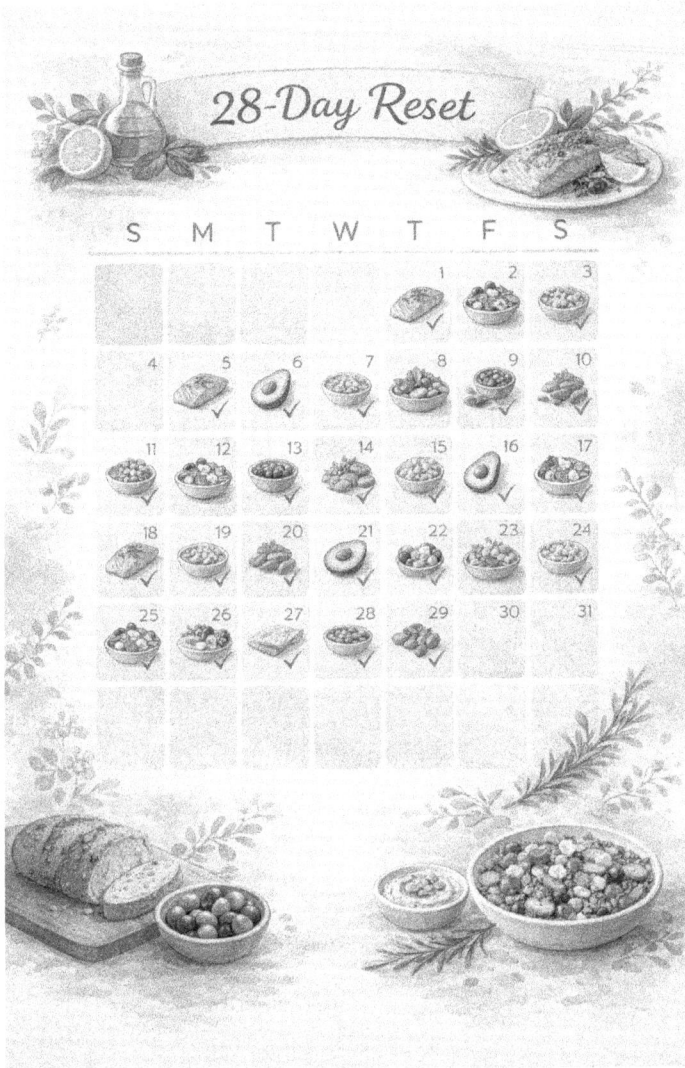

28-Day Reset

Chapter 8

Week 1 — Stabilize & Nourish

Focus: **Blood Sugar Balance, Gentle Digestion, Calming Inflammation**

Week 1 is not about transformation—it's about **reassurance**. Your body has been living on edge, adapting to irregular meals, mixed signals, and background stress. This first week sends a clear, consistent message: nourishment is reliable, urgency is over, and safety is returning.

Everything in these seven days is designed to reduce internal noise so cortisol can begin to settle. If you do nothing perfectly but do these basics consistently, you're doing it right.

What Your Body Is Adjusting

In the first week, your body is recalibrating some very fundamental systems.

Blood sugar begins to stabilize as meals become regular and balanced. This alone can reduce anxiety, shakiness, and the sudden "I need food now" feeling. Digestive enzymes and gut motility start to normalize when meals are predictable and less rushed. Inflammation may begin to soften, which can show up as less bloating, less puffiness, or improved comfort after eating.

You might feel:

- Calmer but slightly tired as adrenaline quiets

- Hungrier than expected as your body tests reliability

- Emotionally sensitive as cortisol lowers and awareness increases

None of this means something is wrong. It means your body is **listening**.

Foods to Emphasize—and Why

Week 1 is about choosing foods that are easy to digest, stabilizing to blood sugar, and anti-inflammatory by nature.

Emphasize:

- **Protein at every meal** to steady energy and reduce cravings

- **Cooked vegetables** for gentler digestion

- **Healthy fats** like olive oil, nuts, seeds, and fish to signal safety

- **Fiber-rich carbohydrates** such as legumes, fruit, and whole grains—paired with protein and fat

These foods work together to slow digestion, prevent glucose spikes, and lower the stress response after meals. You're not eating for excitement this week—you're eating for **grounding**.

This is also not the week to "clean things up" aggressively. If your body has relied on caffeine, sugar, or convenience foods to cope, sudden removal can feel threatening. Gentle substitution works better than force.

Simple Routines for the First 7 Days

The power of Week 1 lies in **repeatability**, not variety.

Anchor your days with a few steady routines:

- Eat within a consistent window in the morning

- Don't skip meals, even if hunger feels mild

- Build each meal around balance, not restriction

- Drink water regularly, especially between meals

- Choose gentle movement—walking, stretching, light mobility

Keep evenings calm. Dim lights earlier. Avoid stimulating tasks late at night. This supports the cortisol rhythm you're rebuilding.

If life feels messy, let food be the stable part.

Emotional Reassurance for Early Changes

Week 1 can bring unexpected emotions. When cortisol drops, the nervous system stops numbing. Feelings that were pushed aside—fatigue, sadness, relief, even grief—may surface.

This is not a setback. It's a **release of vigilance**.

You don't need to analyze or fix these emotions. Acknowledge them. Eat regularly. Rest when you can. Let the process unfold.

Remind yourself:

- You are not doing this to punish your body

- You are not behind

- You do not need to earn nourishment

Safety is built through consistency, not intensity.

What Success Looks Like in Week 1

Success this week is subtle:

- Fewer extreme hunger swings

- A slightly calmer mind

- Meals feeling more satisfying

- Less urgency around food

If nothing dramatic happens, that's actually a good sign. Your body is laying groundwork, not performing.

Week 1 Recipes

Breakfasts • Lunches • Dinners • Stress-Calming Snacks

Theme: Simple, steady, grounding nourishment

Week 1 recipes are intentionally uncomplicated. This is not the phase for culinary ambition—it's the phase for **reliability**. Each recipe is designed to stabilize blood sugar, reduce digestive strain, and gently calm inflammation so cortisol can begin to downshift.

Nothing here requires perfection, tracking, or special equipment. These meals work because they are repeatable, satisfying, and emotionally neutral.

Easy Mediterranean Breakfasts

Goal: steady energy, reduced morning cortisol spikes, fewer cravings later

1. Olive Oil Eggs with Sautéed Greens

Soft-scrambled or gently fried eggs cooked in olive oil, served with lightly sautéed spinach or kale and a slice of whole-grain bread.

Why it works: protein + fat early in the day prevents blood sugar crashes and over-reliance on caffeine.

2. Greek Yogurt with Berries & Nuts

Full-fat plain Greek yogurt topped with blueberries, walnuts, and a drizzle of honey if needed.

Why it works: balanced protein, fat, and fiber support calm focus and digestion.

3. Warm Oats with Almond Butter & Cinnamon

Rolled oats cooked gently, finished with almond butter and cinnamon.

Why it works: warm, slow-digesting carbs reduce stress signaling and are easy on digestion.

4. Avocado Toast with Eggs

Whole-grain toast topped with mashed avocado, olive oil, and a soft-boiled or poached egg.

Why it works: fats + protein slow glucose release and signal safety to the nervous system.

Balanced Lunches

Goal: prevent afternoon crashes and stress-driven snacking

1. Mediterranean Chickpea Bowl

Chickpeas, cucumber, tomato, olive oil, lemon, herbs, and feta (optional).

Why it works: fiber + protein + fat keep blood sugar stable for hours.

2. Sardine or Tuna Plate

Sardines or tuna with olive oil, whole-grain crackers, sliced vegetables, and olives.

Why it works: omega-3 fats lower inflammation and support adrenal recovery.

3. Lentil & Vegetable Soup

Lentils simmered with carrots, onion, garlic, and herbs.

Why it works: warm, grounding, and deeply stabilizing for digestion and energy.

4. Leftover Dinner Plates

Dinner leftovers paired with vegetables and olive oil.

Why it works: predictability lowers cortisol—variety is optional, not required.

Simple Dinners

Goal: nourishment without stimulation; support sleep and recovery

1. Baked Salmon with Vegetables

Salmon baked with olive oil, herbs, and lemon, served with roasted vegetables.

Why it works: anti-inflammatory fats + gentle carbs support overnight repair.

2. Chicken with Olive Oil & Herbs

Simple pan-seared or roasted chicken thighs with zucchini or carrots.

Why it works: protein supports tissue repair; fats promote satiety.

3. Beans & Greens Bowl

White beans or lentils with sautéed greens, garlic, and olive oil.

Why it works: comforting, mineral-rich, and easy to digest.

4. Mediterranean Grain Plate

Quinoa, farro, or brown rice topped with vegetables, olive oil, and protein of choice.

Why it works: carbs without fear support cortisol reduction and sleep.

Stress-Calming Snacks

Goal: prevent cortisol spikes between meals

Snacks are optional—but if hunger or anxiety appears, respond early.
Good options:

- A handful of nuts with fruit

- Greek yogurt

- Hummus with vegetables

- Cheese with whole-grain crackers

- Olives and a slice of bread

Rule of thumb: if you snack, include **protein or fat**—not sugar alone.

How to Use These Recipes in Week 1

- Rotate meals instead of constantly choosing

- Eat before hunger becomes urgent

- Repeat favorites without guilt

- Adjust portions upward if hunger persists

- Keep evenings simple and calming

This is not about eating "light."
It's about eating **reliably enough** that your body stops bracing for scarcity.

Gentle Reminder for Week 1

If food feels less exciting but more calming, that's success.

If your body feels quieter—even slightly—that's progress.

Week 1 is laying the foundation.

The results come later—because safety comes first.

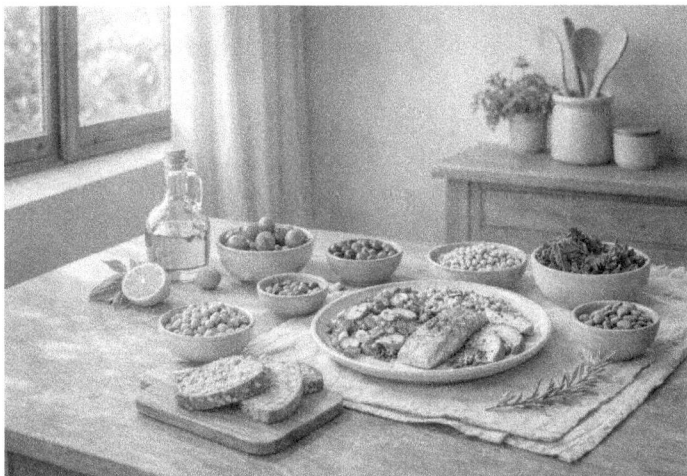

Chapter 9

Week 2 — Calm the Stress Response

Focus: **Adrenal Support, Nervous System Calm, Improved Sleep**

If Week 1 was about reassurance, **Week 2 is about relief**.

By now, your body has received repeated signals that nourishment is steady and danger has passed. Blood sugar is more stable. Meals are predictable. Cortisol no longer needs to stay on constant alert. As a result, the nervous system begins to soften—and this is where many women notice the first meaningful shifts.

This week is quieter than Week 1, but more powerful. You may feel less reactive, less urgent around food, and more able to rest. These are signs that your stress response is finally exhaling.

Why Sleep Starts Improving Here

Sleep rarely improves immediately when cortisol has been elevated for a long time. The body doesn't trust safety after just a few days—it waits for consistency.

By Week 2, several things are happening beneath the surface:

- Blood sugar is steadier at night, reducing adrenaline-driven wake-ups

- Evening cortisol begins to decline more predictably

- Serotonin production improves with adequate carbohydrates

- The nervous system no longer expects scarcity

You may notice it's easier to fall asleep, or that nighttime awakenings feel shorter and less anxious. Even if sleep isn't perfect yet, a subtle sense of *restfulness* often appears.

That's progress. Don't chase it—let it unfold.

Reducing Cravings Naturally

Cravings fade when their cause is addressed—not when they're resisted.

In Week 2, cravings often reduce because:

- Meals contain enough protein to sustain satiety

- Fiber intake feeds gut bacteria and stabilizes appetite hormones

- Blood sugar crashes are less frequent

- Cortisol no longer needs to demand fast fuel

If cravings do appear, they're usually quieter and more informational. Instead of urgency, you may simply feel hunger or a desire for comfort.

Responding calmly—by eating, not negotiating—strengthens trust. And trust is what keeps cortisol low.

Adjusting Caffeine and Meal Timing

This week is a good time to gently observe caffeine's role without forcing change.

Many women naturally find they need less caffeine as energy steadies. If caffeine still feels helpful, small adjustments can make a big difference:

- Eat before or with caffeine

- Delay the first cup slightly after waking

- Reduce late-afternoon intake

Meal timing also matters more now. Eating earlier in the evening and avoiding long overnight fasts can support sleep by preventing nighttime blood sugar dips.

Nothing needs to be rigid. Curiosity works better than control.

Week 2 Recipes

Support calm energy, digestion, and sleep

These meals build on Week 1 with slightly more fiber and variety, while keeping digestion gentle and cortisol low.

Protein-Balanced Breakfasts

Goal: calm mornings, fewer mid-morning crashes

1. Greek Yogurt Bowl with Seeds & Fruit

Greek yogurt topped with berries, chia seeds, and walnuts.

Why it works: protein steadies energy; seeds support gut health.

2. Mediterranean Egg Plate

Eggs with sautéed vegetables, olive oil, and whole-grain bread.

Why it works: early protein reduces cortisol spikes.

3. Savory Oat Bowl

Oats cooked with olive oil, topped with a soft egg and greens.

Why it works: carbs + protein promote calm alertness.

Fiber-Rich Lunches

Goal: sustained focus without afternoon fatigue

1. Lentil & Vegetable Salad

Lentils, roasted vegetables, herbs, olive oil, and lemon.

Why it works: fiber feeds gut bacteria and stabilizes appetite.

2. Chickpea & Olive Bowl

Chickpeas with tomatoes, cucumber, olives, and feta.

Why it works: slow digestion prevents cravings later.

3. Soup + Bread Combo

Vegetable or bean-based soup with whole-grain bread.

Why it works: warmth and fiber calm the nervous system.

Comforting Mediterranean Dinners

Goal: nourishment without stimulation

1. Baked Fish with Potatoes & Greens

White fish or salmon with olive oil, herbs, and vegetables.

Why it works: carbs support sleep; fats reduce inflammation.

2. Chicken & Vegetable Stew

Slow-simmered chicken with vegetables and herbs.

Why it works: deeply grounding and easy to digest.

3. Bean & Grain Bowl

Beans, whole grains, vegetables, and olive oil.

Why it works: mineral-rich and stabilizing for evening energy.

Evening Snacks That Support Sleep

Optional, but powerful when hunger or restlessness appears
Good options include:

- Greek yogurt with honey

- A banana with nut butter

- Cheese with crackers

- Warm milk or dairy-free alternative

- Toast with olive oil

These snacks prevent nighttime cortisol spikes by keeping blood sugar stable.

What Success Looks Like in Week 2

Cravings feel less urgent
Energy is steadier
Sleep begins to feel more accessible
Food choices require less mental effort
If your body feels calmer—even quietly—that's the reset working.
Week 2 isn't about doing more.
It's about letting your body realize it no longer has to guard itself.

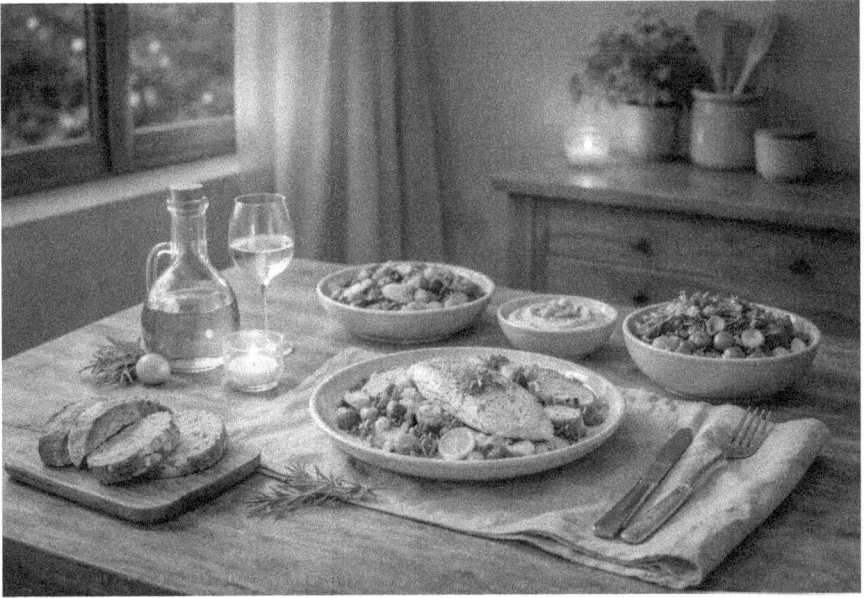

Chapter 10

Week 3 — Release Stubborn Belly Fat Gently

Focus: Fat Loss Without Cortisol Spikes

Week 3 is where many women finally feel a shift—not because they're doing more, but because their body is doing less resisting.

Up to this point, the work has been quiet and internal: stabilizing blood sugar, calming digestion, restoring rhythm, reducing background stress. Now those signals begin to compound. Cortisol no longer needs to guard every calorie. Insulin works more efficiently. Inflammation continues to ease. And when the body feels safe, it becomes **willing**.

This is the week fat loss often feels easier—not dramatic, not forced, but cooperative.

Why Fat Loss Finally Feels Easier

Fat loss becomes difficult when the body perceives threat. High cortisol tells the body to conserve energy, not release it. By Week 3, several protective alarms have quieted:

- Blood sugar swings are fewer

- Meals are consistent and satisfying

- The nervous system isn't scanning for scarcity

- Sleep and recovery are improving

When these conditions are present, the body no longer needs to hold tightly to stored energy—especially around the abdomen, where cortisol receptors are most concentrated.

This isn't about "burning" fat aggressively. It's about **removing the barriers** that prevented fat release in the first place.

What's Happening Hormonally

Hormones rarely change in isolation. In Week 3, cortisol's reduced intensity allows other hormones to function more smoothly.

Insulin sensitivity improves, meaning your body can use carbohydrates more effectively instead of storing them defensively. Leptin and ghrelin—your hunger and fullness hormones—communicate more clearly. Thyroid signaling often feels more supportive as stress demand drops.

For women, especially over 40, this hormonal cooperation matters more than calorie math. The body doesn't respond to pressure. It responds to balance.

Why the Scale May Fluctuate

This is an important moment to reset expectations.

As inflammation decreases, water weight may drop—sometimes quickly. At the same time, increased glycogen storage from eating adequate carbohydrates can temporarily increase scale weight. Both are normal. Neither tells the full story.

What often changes first:

- How clothes fit

- Reduced bloating or tightness

- A softer, less inflamed feeling in the abdomen

- More stable energy

The scale is a blunt tool for a nuanced process. Trust signals, not single numbers.

Trusting Body Signals Again

Week 3 is also about **rebuilding trust**.

You may notice:

- Hunger arriving calmly, not urgently

- Satisfaction appearing earlier in meals

- Cravings becoming optional instead of demanding

- A sense of "enough" without negotiation

These signals are the opposite of willpower. They're cooperation. Listening to them—even when they surprise you—is what keeps cortisol low and progress moving.

Week 3 Recipes

Metabolism-Supportive • Anti-Inflammatory • Satisfying

Week 3 meals are still simple, but slightly more robust. They're designed to support metabolism without stimulation and provide satisfaction without excess.

Metabolism-Supportive Meals

Lemon-Herb Salmon with Olive Oil

Salmon baked with olive oil, lemon, garlic, and herbs, served with vegetables and a whole-food carbohydrate.

Why it works: omega-3 fats reduce inflammation and support fat metabolism.

Chicken & White Bean Skillet

Chicken thighs simmered with white beans, tomatoes, herbs, and olive oil.

Why it works: protein + fiber support steady energy and satiety.

Anti-Inflammatory Ingredients to Emphasize

- Extra-virgin olive oil

- Fatty fish

- Leafy greens

- Tomatoes

- Garlic and herbs

- Legumes

- Whole grains

These ingredients don't force fat loss—they **remove friction** from the process.

Satisfying Portions Without Overdoing It

Portions in Week 3 should feel grounding, not light. If meals leave you searching for something afterward, cortisol rises. Satisfaction keeps it low.

A helpful guide:

- Eat until hunger fades

- Stop when comfort appears

- Trust fullness before heaviness

Your body knows when it's supported.

What Success Looks Like in Week 3

- Less fixation on food

- Subtle changes in body feel

- Improved digestion and energy

- Confidence replacing control

If fat loss is slow but steady—or if it feels easier to *not* interfere—that's success.

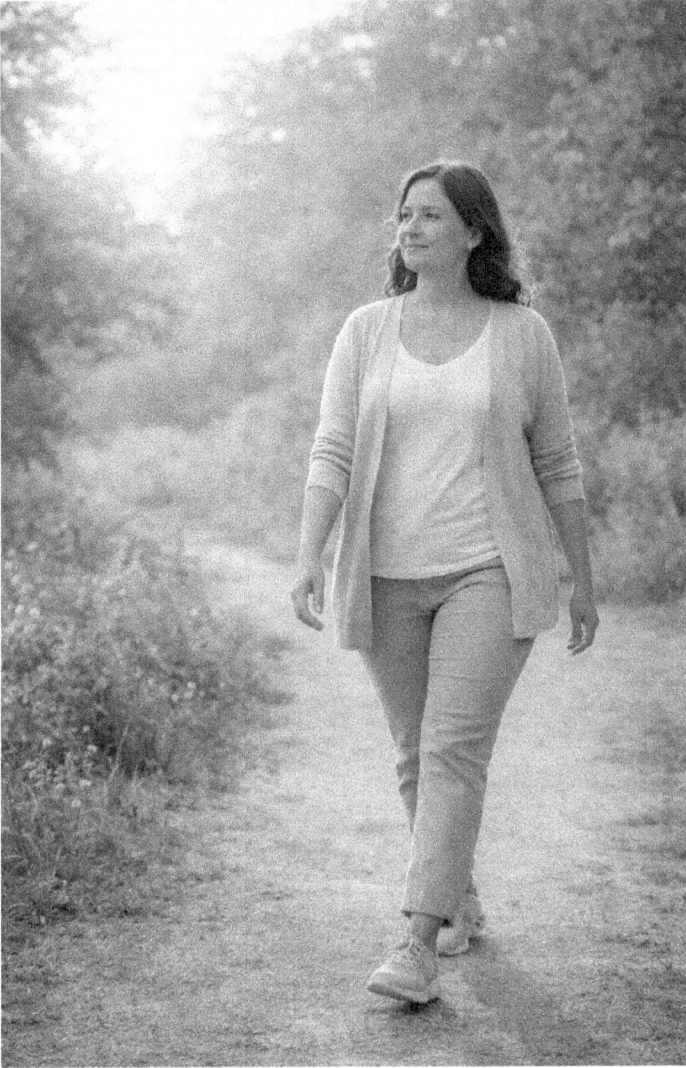

Chapter 11

Week 4 — Restore Energy & Create Momentum

Focus: **Sustainable Energy, Mental Clarity, Routine Confidence**

Week 4 isn't about pushing for more results. It's about recognizing what's already changed—and learning how to keep it.

By now, your body has experienced several weeks of steady nourishment, calmer rhythms, and reduced stress signaling. Cortisol no longer dominates the conversation. Instead of reacting, your system is responding. Energy feels more available. Food feels less charged. Life feels more manageable.

This week is where confidence quietly replaces effort.

Energy Without Crashes

The most noticeable shift for many women in Week 4 is the **absence of dramatic highs and lows**. Energy no longer spikes and collapses. It arrives steadily and lasts longer.

This happens because:

- Blood sugar is consistently supported

- Meals are balanced and predictable

- Cortisol isn't constantly stepping in to "rescue" energy

- Sleep quality has improved, even subtly

Instead of relying on caffeine or sugar to push through the day, you may notice that focus feels easier and fatigue feels more honest. When tiredness appears, it's a cue to rest—not a failure to override.

This is sustainable energy. The kind that supports real life, not just productivity.

Reduced Emotional Eating

Emotional eating doesn't disappear because emotions vanish. It eases because **food is no longer the only regulator available**.

Over the past weeks, you've built:

- Regular eating rhythms

- Balanced meals that prevent urgency

- Emotional neutrality around food

As a result, emotions feel less threatening. When stress appears, the nervous system doesn't immediately demand comfort through food. And when comfort eating does happen, it's calmer, conscious, and guilt-free.

That shift alone lowers cortisol and keeps momentum intact.

Feeling "Normal" Around Food Again

This may be the most important outcome of the reset.

Feeling normal around food means:

- Eating without negotiation

- Stopping without guilt

- Choosing foods without fear

- Trusting hunger and fullness

Food becomes supportive instead of central. It fuels your day rather than dominating your thoughts.

This normalcy is not accidental. It's the result of safety—physiological and emotional—being restored. And it's what allows progress to continue long after the 28 days end.

Week 4 Recipes

Energizing • Balanced • Nourishing • Practical

Week 4 meals are designed to support momentum without adding complexity. They're flexible, repeatable, and easy to carry into everyday life.

Energizing Mediterranean Breakfasts

Goal: clear mornings, steady focus

1. Yogurt with Fruit, Nuts & Olive Oil

Greek yogurt with seasonal fruit, nuts, and a drizzle of olive oil.

Why it works: protein + fat + carbs for sustained energy.

2. Eggs with Vegetables & Toast

Eggs cooked in olive oil with vegetables and whole-grain bread.

Why it works: stabilizes morning cortisol and appetite.

3. Oats with Seeds & Berries

Warm oats topped with chia seeds and berries.

Why it works: grounding carbs that support calm alertness.

Balanced Lunches

Goal: prevent afternoon fatigue

1. Mediterranean Grain Bowl

Whole grains, vegetables, olive oil, and protein of choice.

Why it works: balanced fuel that lasts.

2. Lentil Soup & Bread

Warm lentil soup with whole-grain bread.

Why it works: comforting, fiber-rich, and stabilizing.

3. Leftover Dinners

Dinner leftovers with vegetables and olive oil.

Why it works: predictability keeps cortisol low.

Nourishing Dinners

Goal: recovery and evening calm

1. Fish with Vegetables & Potatoes

Baked fish with olive oil, herbs, vegetables, and potatoes.

Why it works: supports overnight repair and sleep.

2. Chicken with Beans & Greens

Chicken with legumes, greens, and olive oil.

Why it works: satisfying without heaviness.

3. Vegetarian Mediterranean Plate

Beans, grains, vegetables, olive oil, and herbs.

Why it works: mineral-rich and calming.

Smart Snacks for Busy Days

Optional, supportive, pressure-free

- Nuts and fruit

- Yogurt

- Cheese and crackers

- Hummus and vegetables

- Toast with olive oil

These snacks prevent energy dips and emotional urgency when life gets busy.

What Momentum Really Means

Momentum isn't strict adherence.
It's **confidence**.

Confidence that:

- Your body responds to consistency

- Food doesn't need to be controlled

- Stress can be met without punishment

- Progress doesn't require intensity

Week 4 is where you stop "doing the reset" and start **living the rhythm**.

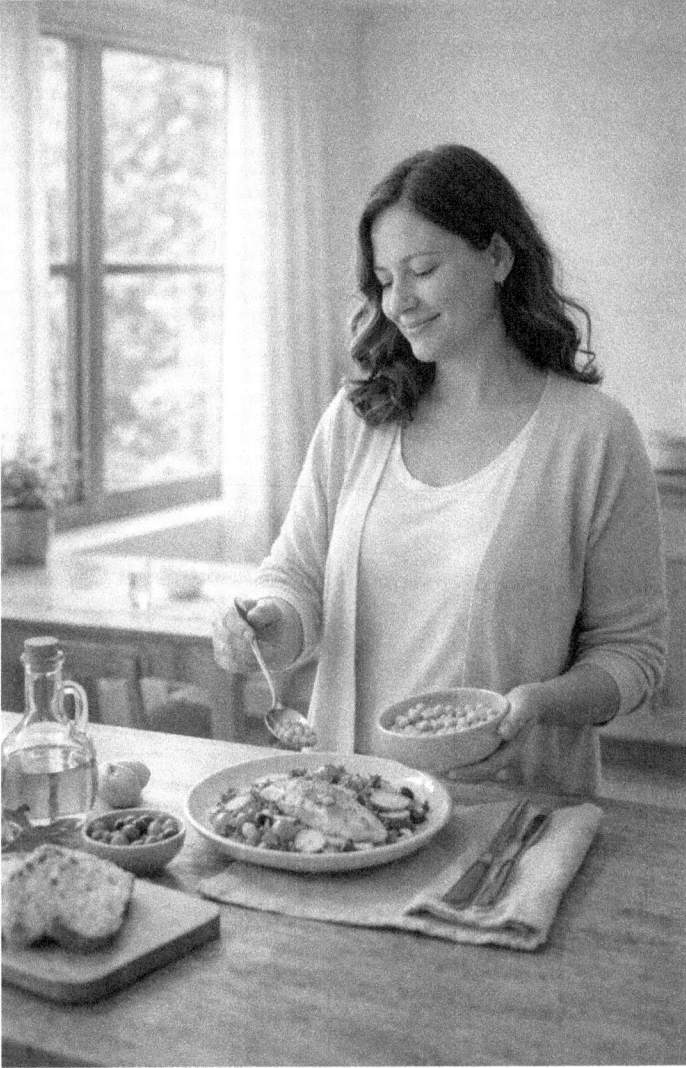

Chapter 12

How to Continue Without Reset Fatigue

The most important thing to understand as you move beyond the 28-day reset is this: **you are not starting over—you are continuing forward**.

Reset fatigue happens when a plan feels temporary, rigid, or disconnected from real life. This chapter exists to prevent that. What you've built over the past four weeks isn't a fragile routine that collapses the moment structure loosens. It's a foundation. And foundations are meant to hold weight, movement, and change.

Transitioning Out of the 28 Days

The end of the reset is not a finish line. It's a **shift in posture**.

Instead of asking, *"What's next?"*, the better question is, *"What already works that I want to keep?"*

As you transition:

- Keep regular meals as your anchor

- Maintain balanced plates as your default

- Let hunger and fullness guide portions

- Allow flexibility without abandoning structure

You don't need to add new rules or tighten control. The reset worked because it reduced stress—not because it demanded intensity. Carry that same principle forward.

If something feels destabilizing, return to the basics you practiced in Week 1. That's not regression. That's maintenance.

Flexible Mediterranean Eating

The Mediterranean approach is sustainable precisely because it allows variation. It's not a meal plan—it's a **pattern**.

Flexibility looks like:

- Rotating proteins, vegetables, and grains based on preference

- Adjusting portions based on hunger, activity, and stress

- Enjoying foods you love without needing to "balance them later"

- Eating simply on busy days and more elaborately when time allows

The goal is not to eat Mediterranean food perfectly. It's to eat in a way that keeps blood sugar stable, inflammation low, and cortisol calm—most of the time.

Consistency beats precision. Always.

Handling Social Meals

Social meals are where old anxiety often returns—not because food is wrong, but because **pressure** returns.

Here's what keeps cortisol low in social settings:

- Eat beforehand if you're very hungry

- Choose foods that feel familiar and satisfying

- Eat slowly enough to notice when you're comfortable

- Stop when you feel complete, not "finished"

You don't need to explain your choices. You don't need to justify stopping. You don't need to compensate later.

Connection lowers cortisol. Enjoying food with others is not a disruption—it's supportive.

Travel and Holidays

Travel and holidays don't undo progress unless they trigger scarcity thinking.

Instead of trying to "stay on track," aim to **stay regulated**:

- Eat regularly, even if choices are simple

- Pair carbs with protein or fat when possible

- Stay hydrated

- Prioritize sleep when you can

- Move gently

You don't need perfect meals on the road. You need predictable nourishment.

When routine returns, so does rhythm.

The Long View

The success of this reset isn't measured by weight loss alone. It's measured by:

- Feeling calmer around food

- Having steadier energy

- Trusting your body again

- Knowing how to course-correct without panic

That's not a reset ending. That's a lifestyle beginning.

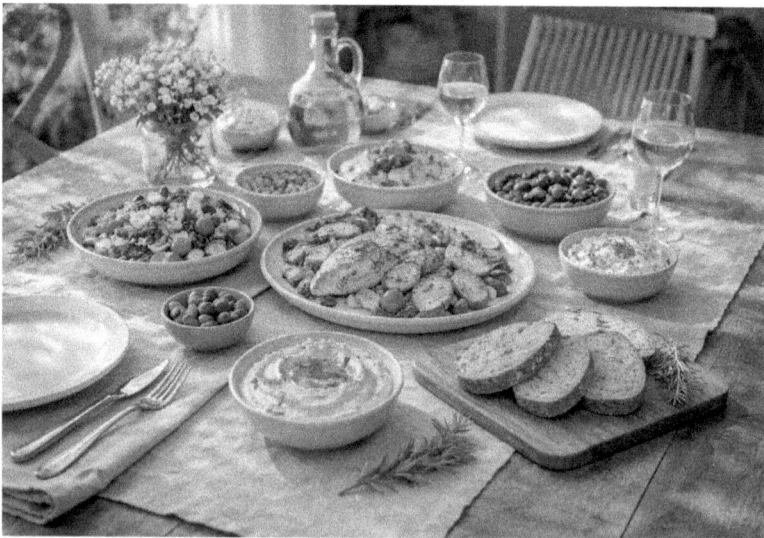

Chapter 13

When Cortisol Spikes Again (And It Will)

No lifestyle—no matter how nourishing—is immune to stress. Life will surge again. Deadlines will pile up. Emotions will run deep. Sleep will get disrupted. And cortisol, doing exactly what it was designed to do, will rise to meet the moment.

That doesn't mean you've failed.

It means you're human.

This chapter exists to remove fear from those moments. Cortisol spikes are not emergencies. They're signals. And when you know how to respond gently, they pass without undoing your progress.

Stressful Seasons

There are times when stress isn't optional—work demands, caregiving, financial pressure, major transitions. During these seasons, the goal is not optimization. It's **containment**.

When life intensifies:

- Keep meals regular, even if they're simple

- Prioritize protein and carbohydrates to prevent blood sugar crashes

- Reduce decision fatigue by repeating familiar foods

- Let movement be supportive, not demanding

Trying to "do better" during high-stress seasons often backfires. The body doesn't need improvement—it needs reassurance. Stability keeps cortisol from staying elevated longer than necessary.

Emotional Setbacks

Grief, disappointment, conflict, and overwhelm don't live only in the mind. They register in the body, often raising cortisol quietly but persistently.

During emotional stress:

- Appetite may change—either increase or disappear

- Cravings may return

- Energy may dip

This is not regression. It's communication.

Responding with restriction or self-criticism amplifies stress. Responding with steadiness shortens its duration. Eat regularly even if hunger cues feel unclear. Choose comforting, familiar foods. Rest more than usual if you can.

Emotional regulation improves when the body feels supported—not judged.

Sleep Disruption

Poor sleep is one of the fastest ways to raise cortisol—and one of the most common experiences in adult life.

Travel, illness, stress, hormonal shifts, or late nights can temporarily disrupt sleep. When that happens:

- Expect appetite to feel less predictable

- Expect energy to feel flatter or jittery

- Expect cravings to be louder

The mistake is trying to "fix" sleep by tightening food or increasing control. Instead:

- Eat consistently the next day

- Include carbohydrates to support serotonin

- Limit overstimulation in the evening

- Accept imperfect nights without panic

Sleep corrects itself faster when cortisol isn't fed by fear.

How to Recalibrate Gently

Recalibration doesn't require restarting the reset or going back to square one. It requires **returning to the basics without urgency**.

A gentle recalibration looks like:

- Three balanced meals

- Optional snacks if hunger appears

- Earlier nights when possible

- Less caffeine, not zero

- Walking instead of pushing

Think of it as lowering the volume—not flipping a switch.

Your body already knows this rhythm. You've practiced it. Returning to it is familiar, not foreign.

The Most Important Thing to Remember

Cortisol spikes don't erase progress. Chronic cortisol does.

What keeps cortisol elevated is not stress alone—it's **how long the body believes the stress will last**. When you respond with steadiness instead of alarm, the spike resolves.

That's resilience.

Not rigidity.

Not perfection.

Not control.

Just the ability to come back to center—again and again.

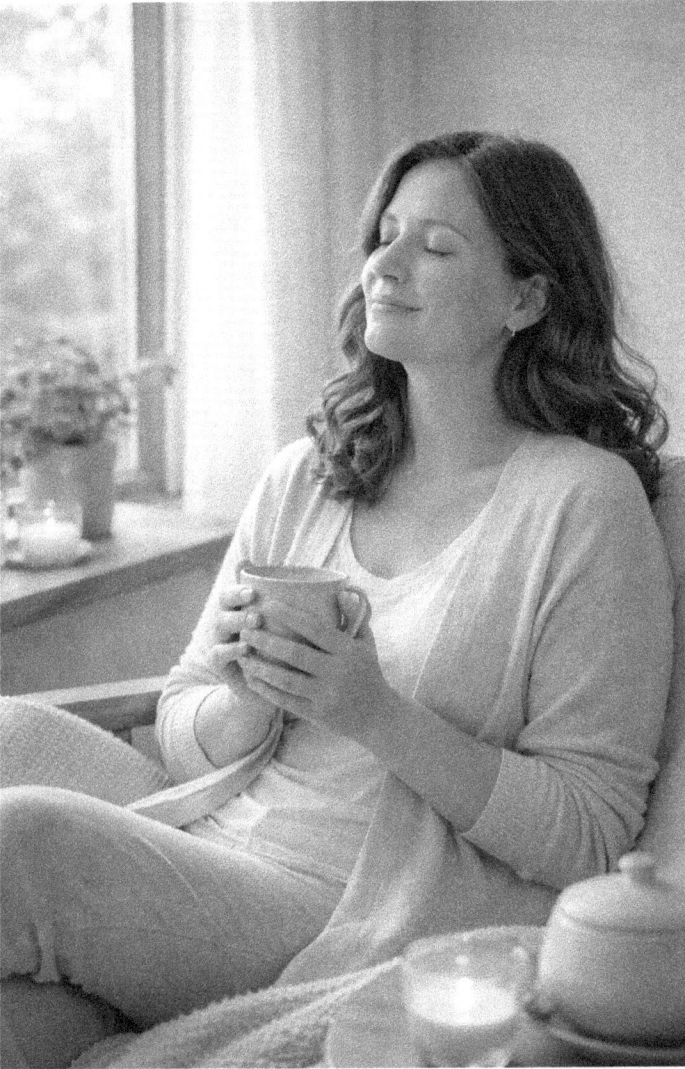

Chapter 14

Your Long-Term Cortisol-Calm Blueprint

What you've built over these weeks is not a fragile balance that disappears without constant effort. It's a new internal baseline—a quieter nervous system, steadier energy, and a relationship with food that no longer feels like a battleground.

This chapter is your blueprint for keeping that baseline intact long after the reset fades into memory. Not through discipline. Through rhythm.

Daily Habits That Protect Hormones

Hormones respond to what you do *most often*, not what you do perfectly.

Daily cortisol protection comes from a handful of quiet, repeatable actions:

- **Regular meals** that prevent blood sugar drops

- **Morning light exposure** to anchor your cortisol rhythm

- **Adequate protein and carbohydrates** to prevent stress signaling

- **Gentle movement** that supports circulation without depletion

- **Intentional pauses**—moments where you stop rushing

These habits work because they are boring in the best way. They reduce decision fatigue. They make your days predictable enough for your nervous system to relax.

You don't need to optimize every morning. You need enough mornings that feel safe.

Weekly Food Rhythms

Weekly rhythms keep you out of reaction mode.

Instead of planning every meal, think in **patterns**:

- A few reliable breakfasts

- Familiar lunches you rotate

- Simple dinners you can repeat

- Snacks available before hunger turns urgent

When food decisions become automatic, cortisol stays lower. The body doesn't feel the need to scan for scarcity or brace for restriction.

Some weeks will be beautifully balanced. Others will be messy. What matters is that your *default* supports stability.

Structure is not rigidity. It's relief.

Monthly Self-Check-Ins

Progress without awareness eventually drifts.

Once a month, pause—not to critique, but to notice:

- How is your energy compared to last month?

- How does food feel emotionally?

- Are cravings louder or quieter?

- Is sleep more supportive or more fragile?

- Where does stress feel highest right now?

These check-ins are not audits. They're conversations with your body.

If something feels off, return to the basics—regular meals, earlier nights, gentler movement. You don't need a reset. You need reassurance.

Redefining Success Beyond Weight

Weight is one data point. It is not the whole story—and often, it's the least interesting one.

Long-term cortisol balance shows up as:

- Energy without crashes

- Calm around food

- Fewer stress-driven cravings

- Better sleep recovery

- Emotional resilience

- Trust in your body

These markers predict sustainable fat loss far more reliably than the scale ever could.

Success is not shrinking yourself.

It's expanding your capacity to live without constant self-management.

The Quiet Power of This Blueprint

This blueprint doesn't promise control.

It offers **cooperation**.

When your body feels safe, it stops fighting you.

When cortisol calms, progress becomes sustainable.

When stress is no longer the driver, health follows naturally.

You are not meant to live in reset mode.

You are meant to live in rhythm.

And now—you know how to return to it whenever you need.

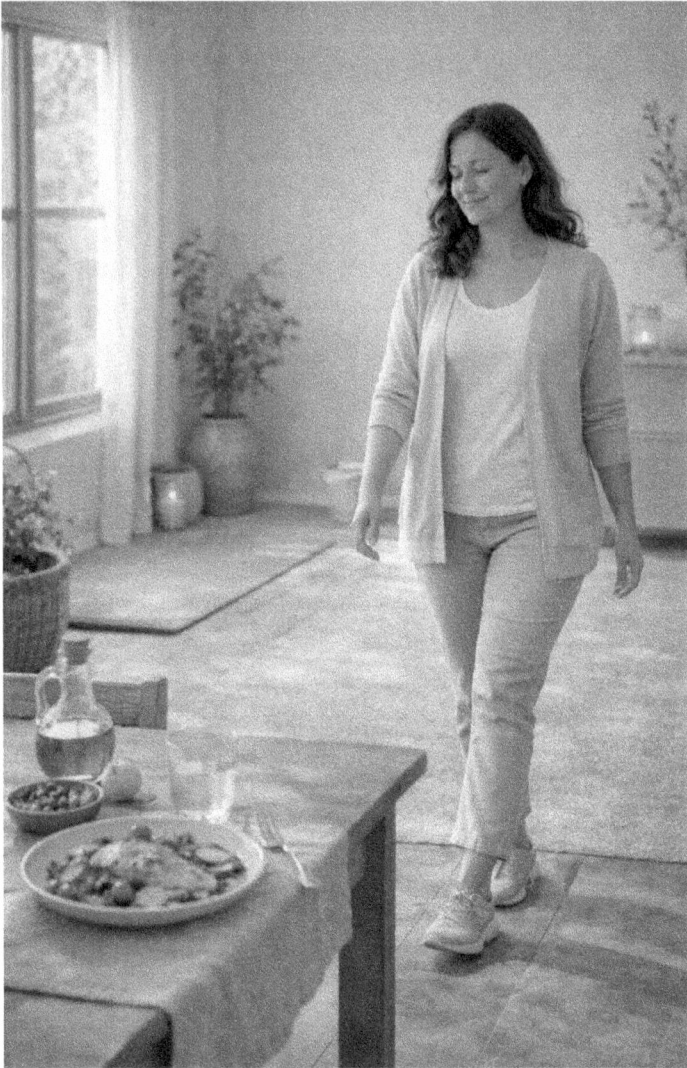

Acknowledgements

I wish to thank the countless individuals—readers, health practitioners, and nutrition experts—who have inspired this work. Your questions, insights, and shared experiences shaped this book into something practical and accessible. Above all, I am grateful to the community of everyday people seeking healthier, more energized lives; your determination proves that transformation is always possible.

9 781685 225278